COUNSELLING
CREATIVE ARTS THERAPISTS

Dr. Geoff Pelham and Jenny Stacey

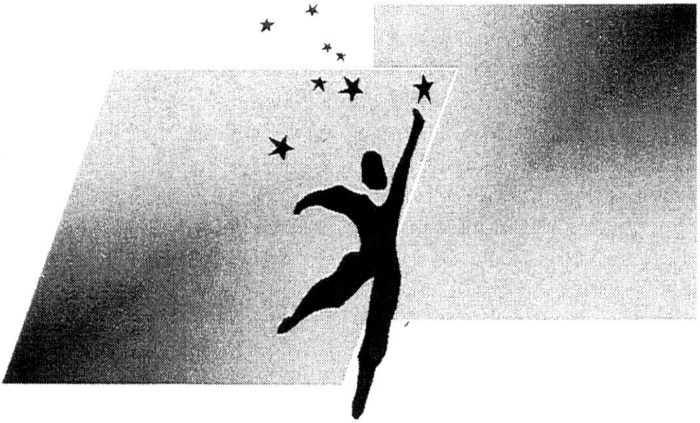

Counselling Skills for Creative Arts Therapists

Dr. Geoff Pelham and Jenny Stacey

Published by Worth Publishing Ltd, 1999

First published in Great Britain in 1999 by Worth Publishing Ltd
Reprinted 2007

ISBN-13: 978-1-903269-00-8

Printed in Great Britain by Grosvenor Group (Print Services) Ltd

Worth Publishing

Contents

Dr. Geoff Pelham is a Senior Lecturer in Counselling at Leeds Metropolitan University, a Counselling Supervisor and a BAC Accredited Counsellor and Trainer.

Jenny Stacey is a State Registered Dramatherapist, Dramatherapy Tutor and Supervisor, and teaches Dramatherapy at the Institute for Arts in Therapy and Education, London.

Introduction

The purpose of this book is to offer an introduction for creative therapists to counselling skills and counselling. Perhaps because of the divisions created by differing traditions in training and professional organisations, it is often the case that people working in related but distinct traditions have little knowledge of each other. There is a great deal of common ground between creative therapists and counsellors. There are also differences in perspectives and key skills. The intention here is to look at these similarities and differences and provide a short introduction to counselling which may prove fruitful to creative therapists.

The first section of the book is a brief discussion of the nature and history of counselling and counselling skills. The approach to counselling adopted in this book is explained. This is followed by an exploration of the relations between counselling and the creative therapies.

In the second section fundamental counselling skills are outlined and discussed. Empathy and congruence are explored as the primary means for engaging with the client's internal and external world.

The third section addresses how the therapist can attend to the client's recreation of his or her own particular "drama" in the therapeutic relationship. The notion of *repeating patterns of behaviour* is introduced, and explored in some depth in relation to the therapeutic frame.

What is Counselling?

Many attempts have been made to define counselling. The British Association for Counselling (B.A.C.) describes it in the following way:

> *"The nature of counselling is to provide an opportunity for the client to work towards living in a more satisfying and resourceful way. The term 'counselling' includes work with individuals, pairs or groups of people often, but not always, referred to as 'clients'. The objectives of particular counselling relationships will vary according to the client's needs. Counselling may be concerned with developmental issues, addressing and resolving specific problems, making decisions, coping with crisis, developing personal insight and knowledge, working through feelings or inner conflict or improving relationships with others. The counsellor's role is to facilitate the client's work in ways that respect the client's values, personal resources and capacity for self-determination."*

(Code of Ethics and Practice for Counsellors; reproduced by kind permission of the British Association for Counselling, November 1999)

This description is very wide and it is likely that many creative therapists would see similarities here with their own practice. It does not, however, offer a very clear definition of exactly what counselling ***is;*** rather it outlines the kind of problems and issues clients bring to counselling, and the counsellor's role in the relationship. Part of the difficulty in providing a clear definition is that there is such a wide spectrum of schools and forms of counselling, ranging from psychodynamic approaches, through the many humanistic schools, to cognitive and behavioural counselling.

This lack of clarity is exacerbated by the difficulties in trying to distinguish between counselling and psychotherapy. To quote the B.A.C. Codes again:

> *"It is not possible to make a generally accepted distinction between counselling and psychotherapy. There are well founded traditions which use the terms interchangeably and others which distinguish them."*
>
> (Ibid.)

Every attempt to find clear-cut distinctions between counselling and psychotherapy has failed. Closer examination of the distinctions indicates that they are rooted more in differences in professional allegiance and status than differences in practice.

The Distinction Between Counselling Skills and Counselling

In the counselling tradition a distinction is drawn between the use of Counselling Skills and Counselling.

> **Counselling Skills** can be used by anyone who wishes to facilitate another person to talk about something. Such skills are additional resources for someone in whatever role she happens to be. For example, a nurse might use counselling skills in a conversation with a patient, as might a teacher with a pupil. Likewise a parent might use such skills with a child (as might a child with a parent!).
>
> **Counselling** involves the use of counselling skills within a formally agreed contract between a person(s) in the role of client and a person in the role of counsellor, stating the conditions under which the parties meet to explore the issues of the person in the client role.

This distinction is reflected in the titles of training courses. There are courses in Counselling Skills attended by a range of professionals (such as doctors, probation officers, teachers, police officers, managers) who wish to develop their interpersonal skills but have no interest in becoming counsellors. Such courses can provide the preliminary training for progression to counselling courses. This preliminary training is sought by people who intend to progress to further training as a counsellor.

At the same time there are courses that provide professional training in counselling. Such courses are more and more seeking accreditation from professional bodies, such as the British Association for Counselling.

A Brief History of the Development of Counselling Skills

Perhaps the most important figure in the development of the counselling skills approach is **Carl Rogers**. During the 1950-60s he developed the **Person Centred** approach to counselling and psychotherapy (it was initially called Non-Directive, then Client-Centred), and the content of most counselling skills courses derive from his work (Rogers, C. 1951; 1961).

In Rogers' view if the therapist held certain *attitudes* toward the client then therapeutic change would occur. If the counsellor truly believes and trusts that the client is the only person who knows what is best for herself, and if the counsellor has *unconditional positive regard,* is *empathic* and *congruent,* then these are the three necessary and sufficient conditions for the client to change.

UNCONDITIONAL POSITIVE REGARD is being absolutely non-judgmental.

EMPATHY is being able to see the world from the client's perspective, and communicating that understanding to the client.

CONGRUENCE is being real and genuine with the client.

Rogers set out what are still seen as the basic personal attitudes for counselling, but others, such as Traux and Carkhuff (1967) argued that *attitudes* are not very teachable, and that these attitudes could be translated into specific *skills* that can be described, taught and practised. Rogers was dismayed that his ideas had been so transformed, where technique began to replace the qualities of the relationship. The parody of his ideas is captured in oft-told stories of how the counsellor simply and mechanically repeats the last few words the client has spoken. Nevertheless, the movement toward the ever more extensive and detailed specification of individual skills gathered pace in subsequent decades. One of the most well know systematic approaches is by **Gerard Egan**, whose book *The Skilled Helper* (1994) is viewed by many as the standard work on counselling skills. In Egan's book the notion of skill is dominant. A person's difficulties are the result of poor personal and interpersonal skills; the remedy is the development of the necessary skills.

Other approaches to counselling such as *psychodynamic* and *cognitive-behavioural* have also, over the years, sought to specify the particular required skills. The pressure to be more and more specific, to define ever more clearly what counsellors should actually ***do***, has been accentuated by movements in education toward clearer definitions of criteria for assessment and judgement, the government supported drive toward competency based training and education (such as NVQs), and the pressures on the counselling profession to be ever more accountable.

The abiding tension throughout this history, which continues to this day, is to what extent is counselling fundamentally about the *qualities of the meeting* (Carl Rogers' position), or the technical *use of skills*.

The Approach to Counselling and Counselling Skills in this Book

It is important to be clear about the perspective on Counselling and Counselling skills that has been adopted for this book. The writers accept the B.A.C description of counselling and work within the psychodynamic and humanistic traditions. It is anticipated that readers are practising therapists who would like to know some of the fundamental counselling skills, but would also value some exploration of the counselling approach to therapy.

We take the concept of ***relationship*** as a central integrating theme.

Relationships are:

- **The crucible for the development of a sense of self and self in relation to others.**
- **At the heart of the problems/issues clients bring to counselling (problems in relations of self to self and self to others).**
- **At the heart of the counselling process itself (the counsellor-client relationship).**

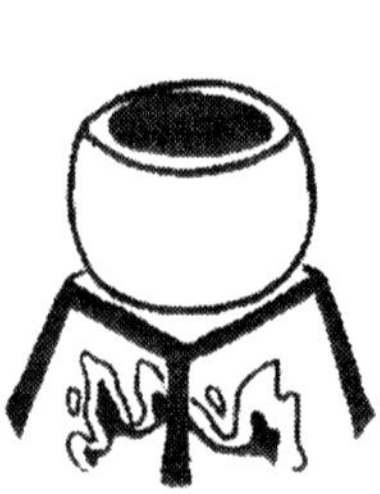

In terms of the debate outlined above, this relational approach assumes that the ***qualities of the meeting*** between practitioner and client are fundamental ***and*** that it is possible and important for the practitioner to develop interpersonal skills that facilitate the meeting.

The tension between these two aspects will always be present. A desire on the part of the practitioner to meet with the client in a genuine and facilitative way may be marred by poor interpersonal skills. On the other hand, a practitioner may use good interpersonal skills to avoid real contact with the client.

Counselling and the Creative Arts Therapies

What are the similarities and differences between counselling and the creative arts therapies?

As we have said, it is likely that many creative arts therapists would view the B.A.C. description of counselling as, at least to some degree, a description of their own practice. Creative arts therapists are familiar with the range of counsellor:client relationships (individuals, couples, groups) There is also the intention to facilitate the client to explore problems/issues within a context of respect for the clients' personal resources and self-determination, and ethical practice.

A primary difference between the traditions may be the ***medium*** through which the form of therapy seeks to effect change. The theory and practice of each particular creative arts therapy is organised around its creative medium. For example, Dramatherapy understands the therapeutic process through the medium of **drama**. In this tradition the concept and technique of "dramatic distance" offers a way of exploring whilst containing powerful emotions. Plays may be used to explore important themes. Clients may inhabit and rehearse different roles and be witnessed by the therapist. Drama may be used to reconnect the client to her creativity. Likewise, the music therapist uses **music and sound** to communicate the essence of emotional experience and to explore the client's rhythms, songs and tempos.

Thus each of the creative arts therapies including art therapy, dramatherapy, music therapy, play therapy and dance and movement therapy draws its theory and practice from the resources of their own tradition.

The medium for the approach to counselling adopted in this book is the ***relationship,*** with the ***counselling relationship itself*** the primary medium for therapeutic change. The precise way the relationship is understood varies across the range of psychodynamic and humanistic theories. For example, as said above, in the Person Centred approach the counsellor seeks to provide the client with a relationship through expressing the ***core conditions*** of unconditional positive regard, empathy and congruence. If the counsellor can do this then the client's own self-actualising processes will be released, enabling the client to find answers to her problems. In the more psychodynamically oriented approaches, the counsellor anticipates that the client will bring her familiar ways of construing and acting in the world into the counselling relationship (*transference*) and this can be explored in the here-and-now of the counselling relationship.

A contrast has been established here between the medium of the creative therapies and the medium of counselling. This contrast is relative, one of emphasis that can perhaps be best understood in the metaphor, from Gestalt psychology, of *figure and ground*. The *figure* is where attention is focused; the *ground* is the necessary context for the figure. Attention can switch so that what was figure becomes ground, and what was ground becomes figure. For example, the figure of my attention may be a book whilst reading. Part of the ground, to which I am not consciously attending, may be the temperature and lighting. If the room grows cold and/or dark, then this aspect may become figure (as I switch on a light and/or turn on a heater) and the book becomes ground. When the heating/lighting is dealt with, the book will again become figure and the environment the ground. Attention switches between figure and ground according to the needs and interests of the person.

Working with this metaphor it may be said that in the creative arts therapies, the medium of the particular therapy, (e.g. drama, art, music or dance) is the predominant figure and the therapeutic relationship the ground. The "figure" for the art therapist will be facilitating the client's exploration of his issues through the theory and practices of art therapy. It may be that the "ground" (the therapeutic relationship) suddenly claims attention: if, for example, the client said he wished to change the arrangements for meeting. When such issues have been dealt with, however, the relationship per se would become "ground" again.

In the relational counselling approach, the relationship is the "figure" and creative techniques the "ground". As indicated above, the attention of the relational counsellor will be on understanding the significance of past and present relational issues for the client, and, most especially, the counsellor will attend to the counselling relationship itself as the primary medium for change. The counsellor may shift focus to consider using various techniques, and may draw upon the resources of the creative therapies (e.g. inviting the client to paint) but the importance of the relationship will still be central. So, for example, the counsellor might ask herself why have I invited the client to paint now? Is it because I am feeling stuck and painting will be something to do to relieve the tension? What may be the effect of using particular techniques? If the client discovers that the medium powerfully facilitates personal material, will this accentuate the tendency for him to view the therapist as an all-powerful person who holds the key to transforming his life?

Words and the Creative Therapist

Creative therapists sometimes describe a tension between the use of their own creative medium with a client and the "ordinary talking" that happens before, between and after its use. It is as if the "real work" happens through the art, dance, music, drama or play, with a somewhat awkward sense of switching back to non-therapeutic talking between time. The counselling skills described in this book offer another possibility. They offer a way of ***translating*** the content and process of the creative medium into the verbal medium and thus ***acting as a bridge*** between the two media, facilitating continuity and coherence. The development of these counselling skills can provide the therapist with more confidence in interweaving the creative and verbal aspects of their work. In the next section, description of the various counselling skills is followed by an example of how the skills may be used through the different creative arts media.

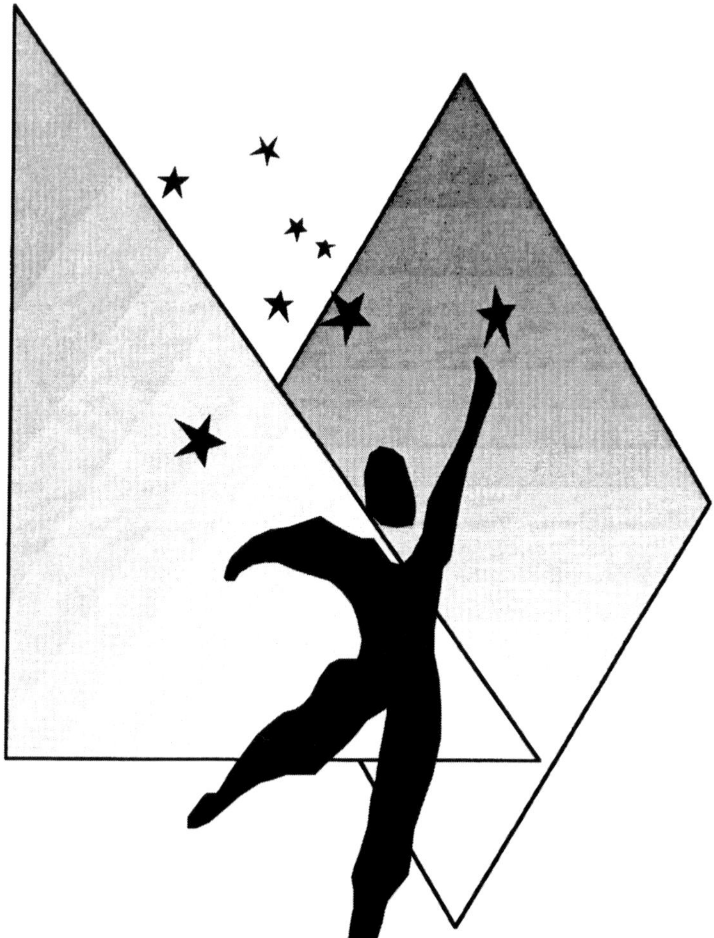

Fundamental Counselling Skills

1. "Just" Being There
2. Facilitating the Person to Tell His or Her Story
3. Attending to Repeating Patterns of Behaviour
4. The Use of the Therapeutic Frame

1. "Just" Being There

The most basic counselling "skill" is the ability to "be" with a person who is distressed and seeking assistance. As simple as it sounds, the ability to just "get alongside" and be with someone in distress is perhaps the hardest thing to do. It can be emotionally difficult and uncomfortable to be in the presence of such a person, to simply hear the distress without seeking to change it, to make it into something else. Almost without exception, if you listen to someone meeting another in distress, such as a parent with a child, the person will seek to take the distress away. The child cries after falling over, the parent says something like: *"It will be better soon"*, or *"I said it would end in tears"* rather than something that catches the child's experience like *"I guess that hurts"* or *"I guess that was frightening"*.

When meeting others in distress people often experience a pressure to "do something" to make things better. We offer advice, minimise the distress, seek solutions, blame someone and so forth. A well-developed professional persona, with accompanying theory and skills, provides additional possibility of ever greater and more sophisticated defences against the discomfort of meeting (Ram Dass and Gorman, P. 1985; Shainberg, D. 1983). It may be easier to offer a diagnosis, expert advice, or explain the causes of the problem rather than tolerate the anxiety of the other person's distress.

The ability to hold a silence, to give good attention, to contain the desire to *do* and simply *be* with the person is utterly fundamental.

Within the context of ***being*** with the person is the ability to facilitate the exploration of issues and difficulties. There is a wide spectrum of skills available to do this. At the heart of these skills is the ability to **"track"** the person, to accompany but not lead, to allow the person to "tell their story" in a manner and pace of her choosing.

Tracking

Tracking involves noticing what is happening within the client at physical, mental and emotional levels, in order to get a full sense of the client as a whole person.

The counsellor maintains acute and relaxed attentiveness. Tiny body movements and flickers of different facial expressions are noted as well as bold gestures. How the client thinks about his or her world, and what form that thinking takes, needs to be followed and understood. The client's changing feelings are observed by the counsellor, and the effect of those feelings on the counsellor are noted.

At the same time as tracking the client, the counsellor or therapist is attending to their own experience and responses at physical, mental and emotional levels. This duality of attention is essential to the counselling process. Tracking need not involve communicating any observations to the client, or it may do.

2. Facilitating the Person to Tell His or Her Story

The skills of **reflecting, paraphrasing**, **focusing**, **empathic responding** and **use of immediacy** are the core skills for facilitating a person to tell her story (with the inevitable paradox that the skills themselves can also be used defensively as a way of avoiding contact).

(a) Reflecting

As the creative therapist knows well, a person can communicate much of his or her experience and patterns of relating without words. However, words and language have their place and due importance. Reflecting words, literally putting back to the client that which has been said, is a basic skill. It may seem simplistic. Its beauty is in its simplicity.

> **Repeating the client's words exactly, with similar emphasis, can convey to the client that the counsellor or therapist is truly listening to them.**

This builds trust. Sometimes it is the first time that anyone has ever paid the client that much attention, or shown that degree of respect. Sometimes it is enough to enable the client to start their story, knowing that their words are not immediately going to be interpreted, changed, intercepted, conflated with someone else's ideas or opinions or simply ignored. Reflecting the last words of someone's sentence back to them, with a mild upward inflection (i.e. with a slight question) can also be a useful way for the counsellor or therapist to establish a solid sense of what is happening for the client, if the work has become very confusing.

So the client might say..."I'm tired"
The reflection would be..."You're tired?"

Or the client might say..."I really love playing this drum, I want to take it home with me"
And the therapist might reflect back..."You really love playing that drum, you want to take it home with you?"

Nothing has been added to the client's words, *nor removed*, so he or she is free to continue, knowing that the counsellor is truly alongside them. Reflecting is best done in short chunks, but the counsellor or therapist will probably find her memory improving over time!

Reflecting and the Creative Arts Media

Reflecting can be used by the creative therapist using his or her own medium.

> John has picked up a tambourine to express himself. He hits it hard, creating a short burst of sound. The therapist also picks up a tambourine and plays back exactly the same sounds. John responds, developing the theme. Again his therapist puts back to him exactly what she has

heard, with no elaboration. This pattern is repeated in a number of cycles as John further expresses himself through sound and rhythm.

(b) Paraphrasing

Paraphrasing is reflecting back to the person the basic details of what was said in a summarised form, including key words. It is a skill that is often used when first meeting a person, when there is little background knowledge of the issues.

For example a pupil may say to a teacher:

"I have not got my homework because my computer with all the stuff on crashed last night and my parents would not help me sort it all out because they are cross with me for staying out late"

A simple paraphrase would be:

"So you have not got your homework because your computer crashed and your parents wouldn't help because they are cross with you"

Relevant details have been picked out from pupil's statement and repeated back to her.

Paraphrasing is a useful intervention to help the other person to say more. In this example:

- The teacher is following what the pupil has said and prepares the ground for the pupil to say more, rather than leading or diverting the conversation (by saying for example, *"why did you leave it so late to print the stuff out?"; "why were you out so late?"; "I am not interested in excuses, it is your responsibility to get the work in").*

- She demonstrates to the pupil that she does want to hear and understand what the pupil has to say

- She checks her understanding of what the pupil is saying. This can be very important if the pupil (or any other person) came in and says a lot very quickly, or gives a great deal of detail. The listener can stop the person by saying something like: *"can I just stop you there to check I understand what you are saying".* This allows the person to assimilate what is being said in manageable chunks and correct any misunderstanding right from the beginning.

- The teacher provides herself with a breathing space to think if the pupil has said something that has put her under pressure for an immediate response. For example, if the pupil had said: *"I have not done my homework because my parents said the school is rubbish and homework is a waste of time",* a simple paraphrase will carry the advantages listed above and also allow the teacher a moment to think and consider what is the best course of action, given the uncertainties and complexities of the situation.

When people are learning paraphrasing or reflecting they often experience it as a somewhat artificial, almost ludicrous thing to do. They imagine the other person is going to turn round and say, *"Yes, that is what I just said".* This has been known to happen, but in the vast majority of cases the other person takes the paraphrase/reflection as an invitation to say more. One way of understanding this is that conversation is about turn-taking: you say what you want to say; I respond (paraphrase/reflect); you develop further what you are saying.

Paraphrasing and the Creative Arts Media

Paraphrasing can be used by the creative therapist using his or her medium.

Carlos has been using two puppets in his work. They are both still on his hands as he speaks to his therapist. It appears to be outside his awareness that whilst he is speaking he is moving the puppets. The therapist may say: "I've been noticing how the puppets have been moving together while you were speaking. Let me show you what they were doing." He then paraphrases the details of Carlos' sequence of hand movements. This allows Carlos to see a summary of his puppets' movements, which may be helpful to him.

Sally has begun to tell her story and gives details about a complex situation. The therapist paraphrases the information by creating a sculpture with chairs in the room:

"Let me see if I understand you. Over here, where this chair is, we have your mother who is in conflict with your sister, who I shall place here. You feel somehow caught between them. I guess placing you here just about catches that, as you say that you feel close to your mother and angry with your sister."

The therapist, by his tone of voice and manner, invites Sally to correct his understanding and positioning of the chairs. As the session develops, Sally begins to use the sculpt by itting on the chairs and gaining a sense of what it feels like to inhabit each position, and then to role play being her mother and sister.

(c) Focusing

The therapeutic process alternates between expansion and contraction, opening up and honing down. The client has begun to relax, open up and tell their story.

Lots of new information has been brought out, and held-back feelings expressed. Now there needs to be some sifting and sorting. Enabling the client to begin to discriminate between the infinite number of ways of exploring or making headway with an issue becomes an important step.

> The skill of focusing is used to facilitate the client to make choices, to prioritise, to identify and work with what is of value to him or her.

A direction will begin to emerge in which he or she wishes to travel. This may deal with the difficulties that brought the person to counselling, or with something else which has taken precedence. Focusing is used whenever the field has become full (or perhaps over-full) of information, feelings, possibilities, options, shifting priorities or open-ended experiences. It can be used within one session or across sessions. Focusing enables the client to think about their experiences, their feelings, and what they are hoping to change.

> Over some weeks, Zahida has been looking at her feelings for her brother, sharing many instances of frustrating encounters and her wish for a deeper relationship. She uses small toy animals, buttons and other objects to represent how she sees what happens between them.

I could ask her:

- How would she like things to be? (Focus on her hopes)
- What does she think of herself within the sculpt? (Focus on her view of herself)
- What does she think she could change? (Focus on her power, or lack of it)
- What does she feel about the sculpt she has made? (Focus on feelings)
- What does she feel about making the sculpt? (Focus on the process of creation)
- How does she feel about sharing it with me? (Focus on our relationship)
- What would she like to do with the sculpt? (Focus on the intra-personal dynamic between Zahida and the relationship represented)

It is clear that there are many choices of focus, each of which could open many doors. The choice of focus is negotiable between therapist and client, and will change according to the aim of the work at any given time.

A key question is of course:

What would the client like to focus on?

Zahida's choices, in the example given above, provide both Zahida and the therapist with a great deal of information about her ability to focus effectively or not.

Avoidance of focusing, keeping things vague and woolly, ("Oh, and another thing"..."Yes, but...") is a way of staying stuck, or of going round in circles. On the other hand, too much focusing can inhibit play and spontaneity. The counsellor needs to be able to use the skill of focusing as a precision instrument and not a sledgehammer.

(d) Empathic Responding

> Empathy is *standing in the shoes of the other person and seeing the world through their eyes.*

Empathic understanding is at the heart of good relationships throughout life. Such connection and communication begins when the infant is first held by parents or primary caregiver (Stern 1985). To be understood by another is perhaps one of the most deeply meaningful experiences we can have. Empathic understanding *does not seek to change anything*; rather it is a deeply human form of contact that says "*yes I am with you, and I truly seek to understand what it is like to be you at this moment*". And paradoxically the experience of being understood can be a powerful stimulus for change.

Carl Rogers had empathy as one of his three core conditions. It has two aspects or moments. There is the active striving to understand what it is like to be the other, to see the world through their eyes. Then there is the act of ***communicating this understanding to the other person***. This second moment is very important. It is not enough to have an empathic understanding. To be interpersonally significant this understanding must be communicated to the other. Most often, but not always, this communication is through the use of words.

A friend comes to me and she is upset. Her eyes are tearful but she sounds angry. She tells me she was driving her car when a man drove close up behind her, staying close for about a mile, then started flashing lights and gesturing for her to get out of the way. When they stopped at some lights he got out and came to her window and was abusive. She kept the window tight shut. He then drove off laughing at her and mocking her.

I could respond to this in many ways. I could say:

"Did you get his number, you can call the police"
or
"What made him so angry; what kind of speed were you doing?"
or
"I hate men like that, they should be locked up"
or
Something like that happened to me last week on my way to work ...."
or
You poor thing, let me get you a drink"

or
Don't let it upset you, don't let him spoil your day"

Responses such as the above are tempting because it is hard to stay with the depth of feeling and distress. Each of these responses would deflect, in one way or another, from the emotional state of my friend.

The empathic response would form as I put myself in her shoes and imagine the events. I imagine the ***shock*** and then ***fear/anger*** to find this person driving so close. I imagine the ***anxiety*** of wondering what is going to happen, what he is going to do, hoping he will go away and ***fury*** that I am being subjected to this. The car stops at the lights and he comes over. My ***fear*** changes to ***terror*** mixed with a deep ***rage*** and ***shame*** that I have kept the window shut and not confronted him. I imagine the ***relief*** and ***humiliation*** as he drives off, gesturing in triumph at me.

As I seek to respond I think, *what is the heart of this*, because there is so much I could focus upon. I notice how she is with me now, struggling with the aftermath of the events. Her anger seems uppermost. I say:

"That sounds terrifying ....you are outraged by him, ***how dare he!"***

I realise the other aspects of her experience are still to be spoken about, especially the feelings of powerlessness and shame, and I am prepared to empathise with these if she chooses to say more.

Empathy is not identification; it is not becoming the other or losing one-self in the other. It is making the imaginative-intuitive leap to understand the world from the other's perspective whilst still being firmly grounded in my own world. Empathy is rooted in a phenomenological orientation: the client's view of the situation is her truth, her experience of existence now. Empathy offers the opportunity to share in and appreciate her truth. Empathic responding com-municates to her my desire to understand her truth and willingness to share it. Rogers insisted that this phenomenological truth was fundamental and he rejected other definitions of truth that practitioners often rely upon, such as diagnosis or interpretation. From his perspective, these other forms of truth are impositions on the person, which undermine her striving for self-determination.

Empathy and the Creative Arts Media

Empathy can be used by the therapist using his or her medium.

> Beatrice has begun to explore some painful aspects of her childhood. The therapist attunes to Beatrice's experience and empathically responds through a story:
>
> "Once there was a princess who lived in a kingdom with a King and Queen. It was a happy

land, full of love and laughter. Then, when the princess was eight years old, the King went to war and was never heard of again. The kingdom lost its warmth and happiness and a deep gloom descended upon the land. The princess felt her grief like a dagger in her heart, but felt that she should not let this show as those in the kingdom needed her to be strong for all to survive."

Theresa has been painting a rough sea, with a small boat in the centre and lots of monsters down in the depths of the sea. Her therapist empathically responds to the scene: "I imagine that the boat must feel very unsafe on that sea, is that right?"

(e) Congruence

A fundamental assumption and moral stance of counselling is to support the autonomy of the client. The individual should find his own solutions, develop his own capacities, and so forth. The empathic stance is a method that supports this fundamental assumption. It rests on the phenomenological position that the client's interpretation of the world is his truth, which should be deeply respected. Empathy explores the subjective experience, the inner world of the client.

A question arises: where is the "other" in this: where is the relationship with another person? If the counsellor seeks simply to be empathic she will, in a sense, disappear as a separate person. Rogers encountered the issue in the development of Client Centred Therapy. Initially he had two core conditions, unconditional positive regard and empathy.

The challenge from clients and commentators alike was the client-centred therapist became like the alter ego of the client; reflecting back the client's world but with no apparent existence of her own. The client, in a sense, cries out: "*Where are you, is there anyone with me?*"

Psychodynamic therapists have their own version of this issue. The psychodynamic stance of neutrality is designed to facilitate the counsellor as a *blank screen* upon which the client projects her internal world. The therapist, as a distinct person, disappears. This creates a profound problem. If the therapist's theory and technique creates a situation where the client only "meets" his own self reflected back (through empathic responding in client centred therapy, or interpretations of projection and transference in psychodynamic therapy), how can the client discover the "real world" of relationship with others?

Rogers introduced his third core condition ***Congruence*** to Client-Centred Therapy and in doing so allowed for the possibility of a real meeting between counsellor and client that would enable the client to experience something/somebody "from the outside".

Congruence means being real in the relationship.

Like empathy, congruence has two aspects. Firstly the counsellor is open to the experience of her self in the presence of the client (be it love, hate, envy, joy, jealousy, delight, thoughts, fantasies etc.). Secondly, she is willing to share her ongoing experience with the client. Rogers says he would like to be **transparent** to his client, allow them to see right the way through him with nothing hidden. Related concepts of genuineness, authenticity and dialogue are at the heart of other humanistic approaches to therapy, such as gestalt.

The introduction of notions of congruence and authenticity immediately raises issues about when, why and how the counsellor is congruent, and what about. What are the guidelines enabling the counsellor to be genuine in a way that facilitates the client rather than simply dumping the counsellor's own unresolved issues on the client? The fundamental point is that the **therapeutic encounter is organised for the benefit of the client**. Congruence should be in the service of that endeavour.

Some simple questions to provide guidelines for the counsellor:

1. What am I experiencing now (thoughts, feelings, actions)?
2. Is this experience new or unfamiliar?
3. What has happened between us, now or recently, that may have produced these feelings?
4. Is this experience persistent and/or familiar with this client?

5. Can I be very specific about my experience?
6. From my knowledge of myself, how is my present experience connected with my own past and in what ways may my own history be intruding?
7. Can I own the experience as ***my experience***, without blaming the other, interpreting the other, and so forth?
8. How can I share my experience in a way that the client will hear as facilitative, not an attack, or a put down, a criticism, and so forth? In other words, how can I speak of my experience with the best chance that it is heard as *an invitation for mutual exploration?*

An example here may be helpful. I am working with a client and my usual experience is of being absorbed in our meetings such that the time quickly passes. Today I notice I am bored (point 1) and clearly this is unusual (point 2). I find myself looking at the clock and dismayed that only twenty minutes has past. The client is talking about what has happened to her during the week and I cannot identify anything that has happened between us to indicate why I am bored (point 3). The feelings persist (point 4) and I realise I have the choice of ignoring my experience or somehow sharing it in a way that is facilitative. I realise that to just say: *"I am bored"* is likely to be heard as critical and put the client, quite understandably, on the defensive. (point 5). I attend more closely to my own experience and realise that somehow I feel out of contact with the client, as if somehow when she speaks to me I am not really touched by her words (point 6). I think this is the heart of the difference today so seek to put this into words. I say:

"Whilst you have been speaking I've noticed something unusual today. I am normally intensely interested in our work together but today I feel different. For reasons I cannot understand I feel quite disconnected from you and struggle to stay interested in what you are saying (point 7*). My hunch is that there is something important here and I wonder what you make of what I've said* (point 8).

Having said this to the client I notice an immediate change. I am no longer bored. I am intensely interested and somewhat anxious at how the client will respond. The client says:

"Well I know what you mean. The thing is, the past few months have been so very painful. In the past few days I've been feeling better and it is such a relief. I'm rather frightened of being here today because I'm scared that talking to you will bring back all the pain again. So I guess I am talking to fill the space more than get into anything".

We now understand the real agenda for the meeting. It would have been quite possible to spend the whole session "filling the space": talking about things that were actually an avoidance of the real issue. The only access to this agenda was the counsellor's persistent feeling of being bored, and taking the risk of somehow bringing this experience into the meeting.

Congruence and the Creative Arts Media

Congruence can be used by the creative therapist using his or her medium.

> Khailda is a Dance Movement Therapist. Her client Paul has expressed himself through movement and then pauses. Khailda has been empathically following Paul and experiences within herself the desire to move in an explosive, powerful way. Such action is a contrast to Paul's movements but feels like a genuine response to him. She risks sharing this movement. Paul laughs and joins her, developing and elaborating her actions.

> In response to Kate's work, the myth of Persephone comes into the therapist's mind. She decides to share this with Kate. She does this in such a way that Kate is able to tell her that it does not fit with her own view, but the therapist's congruent response does allow Kate to become clearer about her story.

(f) Immediacy

> Bringing attention to the moment in the meeting between the client and the counsellor is known as using immediacy.

The counsellor may draw attention to physical, mental or emotional aspects of the encounter, and attempts to be as objective in description as possible.

"I noticed your mouth tightened as you described the interview"
"I noticed a pang of anxiety in my stomach during the silence"
"I notice that this is the fourth time today that you've mentioned the word 'alone'"
"I notice you are holding your breath"
"I am wondering how you felt just now when I said I was going to have a holiday"
"I am wondering what is going through your mind as you look down at the floor"

None of these comments require a response, but they let the client know that the counsellor is fully present and interested in all aspects of their experience. Using immediacy may leave the client feeling exposed, as it has the effect of increasing intimacy, and must be introduced gently over time as the relationship deepens.

3. Attending to Repeating Patterns of Behaviour

Based upon the experiences from within the crucible of early family and later social life, people organise their approach to life and ways of relating to others into patterns that seem to offer the best compromise between desire and danger. Some aspects of these patterns may be available to conscious thought whilst other aspects may be deeply unconscious, consisting of thoughts, feelings and fantasies that profoundly structure relations with others.

These aspects may be unconscious because they were formed at a very early age before words were available, and/or because they seem potentially dangerous to the self and to established relationships. These patterns are often organised as "dramas": repeating sequences of relating to self and others over time. They tend to become self-fulfilling, creating and reinforcing the difficulties and issues the client brings to counselling. For example, a person may have very little self-confidence and believe others are always critical of him. He readily hears any comments by others as criticism, even when they are not so intended. Consequently he responds in a distancing and attacking way. Other people, in response, become critical and attacking.

Counselling and therapy are usually about attending to these dramas (patterns) in a more or less explicit way, with the intention of transforming them into productive and fulfilling forms of relating.

For the client the counselling or therapeutic relationship is basically a relationship like any other. The client will bring their unconscious pattern of relating into counselling, and this is what a relational counsellor calls ***transference.*** The counsellor will experience the interpersonal effect of the transference, and this forms part of ***counter-transference.*** The dynamics of transference and countertransference have enormous therapeutic potential. Through this process clients not only talk about their difficulties as they experience them in their daily lives, they bring these very difficulties into the counselling relationship. If the counsellor is willing and able to work with the counselling relationship then there is the potential for the client not only to talk about but also to ***re-experience*** their relational difficulties, with the possibility of developing new forms of relating. Taking the example from above, this client will be vigilant for anything that can be understood as criticism by the counsellor, and respond in attacking and critical ways that put distance between the two. There is considerable potential for change if the counsellor can explore with the client what is actually happening between them.

A practitioner, thinker and writer of great importance for both creative therapists and counsellors is D. W. Winnicott. Much of his focus was on relationships, especially the relationship between parent and child, and between therapist and client. He was intensely interested in the paradoxes created by the inextricable links between the development of the sense of self and relations with others. He spoke of *the separation that is not a separation but a form of union.*

He sought answers to these paradoxes in the relation between the inner and outer world of the person. Both realms are crucially important. The truly alive person, the person living a *true self* and not a *false self* is the person who can creatively engage with the external world.

Winnicott focused his attention on what he called *transitional space and transitional objects.* These are spaces and objects that exist in the real world but which have been transformed through the creative subjectivity of the person. A painting is formed from real materials (paper, paint, paint brushes, etc.) and the subjectivity (imagination, artistic talent) of the person. The painting is not solely of one or the other, either the external or internal world. It is of both.

Winnicott believed that therapy is about the creation of a *transitional space* and that the therapist should allow herself to be used as a *transitional object* through which the client will play with his experience and seek to remedy earlier developmental hurt and damage (Winnicott 1971). The client will seek to creatively recreate circumstances that reproduce early trauma in the hope of a different outcome. Put in psychodynamic language, the client will reproduce in the transference the circumstances that mirror earlier trauma, in the hope of a different outcome, a new healing experience. If this transforming experience is to have a good outcome the counsellor must, paradoxically, allow herself to be used by the client so that the circumstances are genuinely recreated. At the same time, she needs to be able to gain an understanding of the process to ensure the trauma is not reproduced in the therapy. The true therapeutic disaster is if the trauma is simply reproduced. This process can be hugely challenging to the counsellor, as the recreation of events can feel **very real** and provoke genuine, deep and often distressing feelings (Casement 1990). It may pose actual, indeed real-world dilemmas. For example, a client who has experienced people being untrustworthy might leave a session alluding to the fact that he may commit suicide. The therapist is left in a state of anxiety and uncertainty: should she break confidentiality and inform the client's doctor of the situation, knowing that to do so would be experienced by the client as a betrayal?

A paradox for Winnicott is that the person's creativity can only emerge from the appropriate *facilitating environment,* especially early in life. Failure to meet the developmental needs of the child, through various forms of impingement, results in premature attention to reality and the creation of a *false self* which adapts to reality rather than creatively *transforming* it.

Winnicott thus has important things to say to both the relational counsellor and the creative therapist. He said that therapy is a form of play, mutual play between therapist and client. A person unable to play cannot be a therapist. The task of therapy is to enable the client to begin to play again. Creativity is the essence of being truly alive, rather than just living in compliance to the dull brute facts of existence.

From Winnicott's work, then, the counsellor is alerted to the likelihood that the client will "use" the counsellor and the counselling set-up, will "play" with it, to creatively recreate important experience. The counsellor can get some understanding of this process for a client if she attends to the client's typical ***repeating patterns of behaviour***, and how the client uses the therapeutic frame to express deeply unconscious aspects of his or her relations with others.

Skills for Exploring Patterns

Some of the "tools" for enabling the client to understand their relational patterns have been discussed above.

> **Empathic responding** enables client and counsellor to understand the client's thoughts, feelings and actions, and also how the client interprets the thoughts, feelings and actions of others. The repetitive patterns of relating often become clear in this process.
>
> **Congruence** enables the counsellor to address the experience of being with the client and perhaps draw attention to, and disrupt familiar patterns.

For example, in the discussion above of congruence in which the counsellor was bored, it might be that an aspect of the client's pattern is to unconsciously avoid saying things that might upset the other (*"I don't want to be here today because I am feeling good and talking to you may spoil that"*). The counsellor's congruent response draws attention to this aspect of the client's pattern. From this it may be that the client can develop different ways of behaving in similar situations, and try out these different ways in the comparative safety of the counselling relationship.

Exploring Patterns and the Creative Arts Media

Creative therapists can use their own medium to explore the repeating patterns of the clients.

> In sessions with his client Joe, Max, a movement therapist, often feels full of sadness at what has happened to Joe during his childhood. In supervision Max is asked to take on the role of Joe and, using movement, show the supervisor how Joe relates to him. By doing this Max sees more clearly how Joe repeatedly pulls him from his "place" as therapist to fulfil his desire for a nurturing father. Moving in this way illuminates what is happening at times in the therapy and allows Max to bring this pattern into their work together.

4. The Use of the Therapeutic Frame

A primary site for the expression of relational dynamics is the **therapeutic frame**. It is a prime site because at first glance it appears to have little or nothing to do with the actual therapy or counselling, and is therefore a "safe" place to express inexpressible things.

When a client comes to the initial assessment session wanting counselling or therapy the therapist and client agree a contract which specifies the agreed conditions for working together.

The therapeutic frame is the contract that 'holds' or contains the therapeutic or counselling relationship.

The frame involves such matters as the forms of intervention (not advice giving, instructing, etc.), time, length, frequency, place of meeting, confidentiality and fees. At one level this agreement can be seen as purely "administrative", creating the necessary arrangements for the work. It can also be seen as an agreement entered into freely by both parties which respects and enhances the autonomy of the client. The client clearly knows and can negotiate the arrangements and can take an informed judgement as to whether or not to enter counselling or therapy. Clear "administrative" arrangements and respect for the autonomy of the client are essential elements of the therapeutic relationship. From this perspective a contract once agreed can be easily changed by mutual agreement.

For example, changes in time or frequency could be made to meet the needs of either party.

The contracting process as described above takes place at a rational conscious level. It is a description that is in some senses formal and abstract, missing some of the important dynamics of the meeting. The relational approach presumes that relationships have both conscious and unconscious components. These components are rooted in the cultural/personal experience of both parties, so that right from the first contact dynamics of class, gender, race, sexuality, disability and family will enter into the therapeutic relationship and affect the management of the frame.

Both parties bring their conscious and unconscious hopes, fears, desires, and conflicts to the meeting which stem from their cultural/personal history. The therapeutic frame will come to embody and be the site for expression of these feelings. From this perspective, the appropriate awareness and management of the frame is fundamentally important for therapy. It becomes the structure within/against which previous experience and expectations around issues of power, authority, safety, containment, desire, anxiety and so forth, are evoked. It is an important place for the creative expression of the client's underlying hurts and hope for healing.

Power and Authority

The frame is the place where the dynamics of power and authority are likely to be most prominent in counselling or therapy. The frame establishes boundaries that can be experienced (by both parties) as enabling through the creation of a "secure base". A secure base is a place of safety from the dangers of the world, a place that eases anxiety, contains fears and is a springboard for exploration. The very security expressed in the firmness of the arrangements can be experienced as an expression of love and caring. The secure base is a product of the reliability, stability and protection from the intrusions of the outside world (through, for example, the agreement about confidentiality that ensures others are "outside" and will not intrude "inside" the counselling relationship). The frame can express and offer all the promise of **good authority,** that is, the positive use of power that is creative and enabling. The absence of good authority can be as destructive as the abuse of power (Pitt-Aikens T & Ellis T.A 1990).

The secure base can also be experienced as reproducing negative experiences of power and authority. It can be experienced as a place of arbitrary imposition of arrangements for the benefit of the person with power (the therapist or counsellor). This can generate feelings of rage, helplessness, rebellion and so forth. The client can come to experience the counsellor's firmness around the frame as a lack of caring (*"if you really cared for me, you would change the time of our meeting/ reduce the fee/ change to meeting twice a week/ write to the Housing Office to help me get a new home......"*). All the client's experience around authority can be replayed in relation to the frame.

The therapeutic frame provides a site for re-experiencing issues of power and authority in both their positive and negative dimensions. And of course (to make things more confusing) the frame may be experienced **in both positive and negative dimensions at the same time**. It can be experienced as offering a secure base and as arbitrary and self-serving.

The frame can also be the site where cultural dynamics of power become most focused in the therapeutic relationship. Relations of class, gender, sexuality, race, disability and so forth are saturated with issues of power. The counselling injunction to offer "unconditional positive regard" is likely to drive out of consciousness these cultural power dynamics.

> The more they are rendered unconscious, the more effect they are likely to have, which will influence the management of the frame.

Containment

The client often comes to counselling or therapy with conscious and unconscious beliefs that certain aspects of his/herself are unacceptable and unmanageable. The unconscious hope may be to find someone who can contain (and thus make acceptable and manageable) these aspects of the self.

The frame is a crucial site for the containment and "holding" of unacceptable/unmanageable aspects of the self. The counsellor's ability to hold the frame when the client is expressing what seem to be unmanageable feelings can be a message to the client that *"I know these feelings are difficult, but I have confidence that in fact you can manage them*". Such confidence can offer the client the holding and containment needed to manage the feelings.

The counsellor's or therapist's inability to hold the frame by, say, offering advice, referral to other agencies, offering extra sessions, going over time, may be an expression of the counsellor's belief that feelings are not containable within the usual frame. The client is likely to understand this communication and this can reinforce the sense of danger and anxiety. So, for example, the counsellor may see the client in great distress at the end of a session and say *"I can see it is hard for you; maybe we could meet again later this week?"* This can seem like a sympathetic and helpful intervention (and in some cases it may be just that) but it is also likely to convey the implicit message to the client: "I don't think you can cope until next week, the feelings are too unmanageable".

Why should the behaviour of the counsellor be so important here? A person's sense of what is acceptable/manageable comes from their history of relations with others. What is acceptable and manageable is often a reflection of **what others have found acceptable and manageable.** If important others have found feelings like anger, or jealousy, or rage, or anxiety unacceptable then the client will have learned that lesson and try to suppress or otherwise avoid such feelings and behaviours. The client will be alert to how the counsellor deals with emotionally laden situations and draw conclusions as to what is safe and acceptable, and what is not.

Why do Therapists Inappropriately Change the Frame?

Pressures to change the frame can come from the client, the therapist and third parties (people outside the therapeutic relationship such as colleagues, other professionals, family/friends of the client).

1. Pressures from the Client

A client may have real and compelling reasons for changing the frame (e.g. a new job that makes the agreed time difficult). At the same time the client may re-experience and replay their own "drama" in the therapeutic relationship, and the very requests and pressures to change the frame can be the re-enactment of their lifelong repetitive conflict and issues. The frame is a particularly important site for the re-enactment of the most unconscious aspects of the drama. The client (and often the therapist) is usually only conscious of the "administrative" side of the frame so that unexpressed conflicts and issues are displaced onto and expressed through the frame. For example, missed sessions may be the result of unacknowledged anger or fear of dependency. Repeated requests to change the time, frequency or fee may express the client's experience and desire/fear of a secure, predictable, reliable relationship.

> The client may also use the frame to prompt the therapist to experience dilemmas that are central to the client's life, but cannot be spoken about.

For example, the client may say s/he can only continue meeting if the appointments are moved to a time that is inconvenient for the therapist. The unconscious agenda may be *"if you really cared for me, you would attend to my needs and not your own"* which might be the dilemma the client experienced as a child. Or again, the client may repeatedly put pressure on the therapist to act inappropriately *("please can we continue working together whilst I also see another counsellor, as it is helpful to get two views"; "I'm about to start a new counselling training course, will you act as a reference as you know me so well").* The client may be attempting to unconsciously communicate his/her experience of being pressured to act inappropriately. **There may also be another unconscious hope: that the therapist will experience the full force of the dilemma and "survive it", that is, find a way of relating that allows both parties to maintain and enhance their integrity**.

In the first example, it would be important for the therapist to carefully attend to the inconvenience that would flow from rearranging (with all the attendant bad feeling that generates) and say that s/he is not in a position to change. Such a response might allow the client to get in touch with the underlying issues as s/he experiences someone who is not going to "sacrifice" him/herself to prove their caring for the client. In the second example it would be important for the therapist to realise that to agree to the requests would be to collude in inappropriate behaviour and again by the therapist turning down the requests the client has the opportunity to more deeply understand the issues.

2. Pressures from the Therapist

The therapist or counsellor may wish to initiate changes to the frame. If the frame is seen as simply an administrative arrangement, then the therapist may see little significance in asking the client to make changes to suit the therapist's needs.

The counsellor may be aware of the importance of the frame and still initiate changes. This happens most often when the dynamics of the counselling relationship stimulate strong feelings in the counsellor. The concept of **projective identification** is important here (Casement 1985; Gray 1994). The client may project into the counsellor feelings or aspects of the self that seem dangerous or unmanageable. For example, a client may experience and project into the counsellor feelings of intense anxiety. The counsellor feels intense anxiety, which affects her/his behaviour (e.g. going over time; offering extra sessions; offering advice; referring the client to another professional). The dynamics here are again closely related to the replaying of the client's "drama" in the counselling.

The therapist will bring her/his own relational history into the work and unresolved issues may lead to changes in the frame. The therapist may need to be liked, to be seen as caring, or be scared of conflict, anger and so forth. The client may unconsciously remind her/him of particular significant people from the past (typically mother, father, sibling) where there are still strong feelings. Such feelings may make it very hard to hold the frame and the therapist may even initiate changes that the client has not requested *("Do phone me at home if you get upset")*.

Unresolved feelings around cultural issues may impact on the counsellor's ability to properly manage the frame. A white counsellor with unexplored feelings around race may act from a pervading sense of guilt and fear of his/her own racism and be overacommodating to requests to change the frame. A middle class counsellor may doubt the ability of a working class client and express this by suggesting a low fee to "help" the client.

What most often happens is that **the client is unconsciously aware of the counsellor's or therapist's unresolved conflicts and draws upon these in the expression of their own drama.**

3. Pressures from Third Parties

Sometimes people outside the counselling relationship seek to influence, or want information about, the counselling. Other professionals (doctors, social workers, probation officers, teachers etc.) believe the counsellor or therapist should know something about the client, or they wish to know something, or they wish to influence the form/content of the work. Relations and friends may have similar agendas. These others may contact the counsellor by phone or letter, and sometimes the client may bring the request into the session *("My doctor/psychiatrist/partner would like to know ....thinks you should know that ....")*

Such requests can put considerable pressure on the therapist. To turn down such invitations to break confidentiality can be viewed by others as unhelpful, obstructive and so forth. If the requests come from high status professionals, this may generate considerable anxiety in the therapist.

To Change or Not to Change the Frame

Unfortunately there is no simple answer to the question of whether it is appropriate to agree to changes in the frame. Judgements have to be made within the context and dynamics of any one particular relationship, at any given time. One thing is certain:

> Changes in the frame will always convey meaning to the client

This meaning can only be understood within the developing relationship. One client may experience counsellor firmness around the frame as communicating care and concern for the client, and a willingness to confront the latter's anger without collapsing or retaliating. A different client may experience such firmness as reproducing parental disregard for the needs of the child, with resulting hopelessness and withdrawal (notice that such a reaction, if explored in the counselling, could be an important source of new insight and change). For such a client to ask for and receive flexibility could be a crucial new experience.

Some guidelines for working with frame issues (highlighting the skills and awareness required)

- Be aware that requests (from whatever party) for changes in the frame carry both conscious and unconscious meanings. Issues arising around the frame may be an enactment of the client's drama.

- Be willing to reflect on your own experience raised by the frame issues. Your immediate response will give you invaluable material for understanding the "drama" being enacted. This may offer you some understanding of how to act. You will need to consider whether your own unresolved personal issues are involved, and whether telling the client about your response will be helpful to him or her.

- Be aware that whatever course of action is taken involving the frame will carry important unconscious meaning and affect the subsequent dynamics of the relationship.

- Whenever possible, do not make sudden decisions about the frame (prompted either by the client's anxiety, or someone else's, or by your own need to please or to fend off hostility.

- Create some space to reflect upon decisions and, where possible, explore the issue with the client. Space can be created in a number of ways, for example simply by not responding immediately to the request but waiting to see what happens next (e.g. the client may make "displaced" comments about how the firmness of other people has been helpful in the past). Saying that you need time to think – and to be able to think together – about the request is congruent, validating and invites the client to join you in recognising the significance of the proposed change. Ideally, suggestions of alterations in the frame can be discussed in supervision.

- Changes in the frame are always an important topic for supervision, as are requests to change the frame of supervision itself. This is especially the case if you find that you are requesting changes in response to something happening in the piece of work you want to take supervision (for example, noticing that you suddenly want to contact your supervisor in between sessions on an issue).

- Dealing with unresolved issues played out around the frame can be disturbing and unsettling for the client and the therapist. You will need courage, alertness, tenacity and quite possibly support to stay with the process. The results, however, can be extremely enriching and constructive; for the client, in his or her journey toward "living in a more satisfying and resourceful way", and for both client and therapist in a shared sense of a more trusting and intimate relationship.

Conclusion

This book has very briefly covered considerable ground. Our hope is that it will provide the creative therapist with new skills and a broader understanding as she switches attention between her own particular creative medium and the therapeutic relationship. Within the therapeutic relationship both parties can use their awareness of what is happening between them to shed light on the client's patterns of relating, and how the client creatively recreates her familiar hurts, longings and desires. These patterns are clearly illuminated around the therapeutic frame.

Integrating relational counselling skills into her repertoire can enable the creative therapist to develop new ways of using her own medium to fruitfully explore the unfolding dynamics of the relationship with her client.

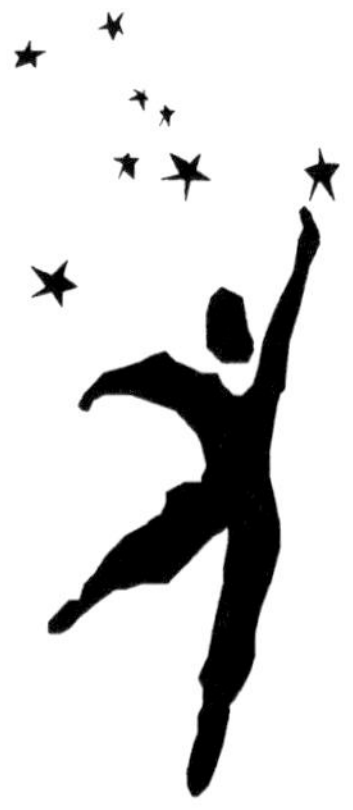

References

British Association for Counselling *Code of Ethics for Practice for Counsellors*

Bowlby, J. *A Secure Base*
Arrowsmith, 1988

Casement, P *On Learning from the Patient*
Tavistock, 1985

Casement, P *Further Learning from the Patient*
Tavistock, 1990

Egan, G. *The Skilled Helper*
Wadsworth, 1994

Gray, A *An Introduction to the Therapeutic Frame*
Routledge, 1994

Pitt-Aikens, T. & **Ellis**, T.E. *Loss of Good Authority*
Penguin, 1990

Ram Dass & **Gorman**, P. *How Can I Help*
London, Rider, 1985

Rogers, C. *Client Centered Therapy*
Boston: Houghton Mifflin, 1951

Rogers, C. *On Becoming a Person*
Boston: Houghton Mifflin, 1961

Shainberg, D. *Teaching therapists to be with their clients* in
Westwood, J. (ed.) *Awakening the Heart*
Colorado, Shambhala, 1983

Stern, D *The Interpersonal World of the Infant*
Basic Books, 1985

Traux, C.
& **Carkhuff**, R. *Towards Effective Counselling and Psychotherapy*
Aldine, 1967

Winnicott, D. W. *Playing and Reality*
Tavistock, 1971